The Let's Talk Library

Let's Talk About When Someone You Love Has Alzheimer's Disease

Elizabeth Weitzman

The Rosen Publishing Group's
PowerKids Press
New York

Published in 1996 by The Rosen Publishing Group, Inc.
29 East 21st Street, New York, NY 10010

Photo credits: Cover photo by Maria Moreno; p.12 by Kyle Wagner; p.15 © Stan Pak/International Stock; all other photos by Maria Moreno.

First Edition

Weitzman, Elizabeth.
      Let's talk about when someone you love has Alzheimer's disease /
Elizabeth Weitzman.—1st ed.
          p.   cm.
      Includes index.
      Summary: Discusses the devastating effects of Alzheimer's disease
and offers basic mechanisms for coping with a loved one's illness.
      ISBN 0-8239-2306-1
      1. Alzheimer's disease—Juvenile literature. [1. Alzheimer's disease.
2. Diseases.] I. Title.
RC523.2.W45 1996
618.97'6831—dc20   95-50794
                                                         CIP
                                                         AC

Manufactured in the United States of America

Table of Contents

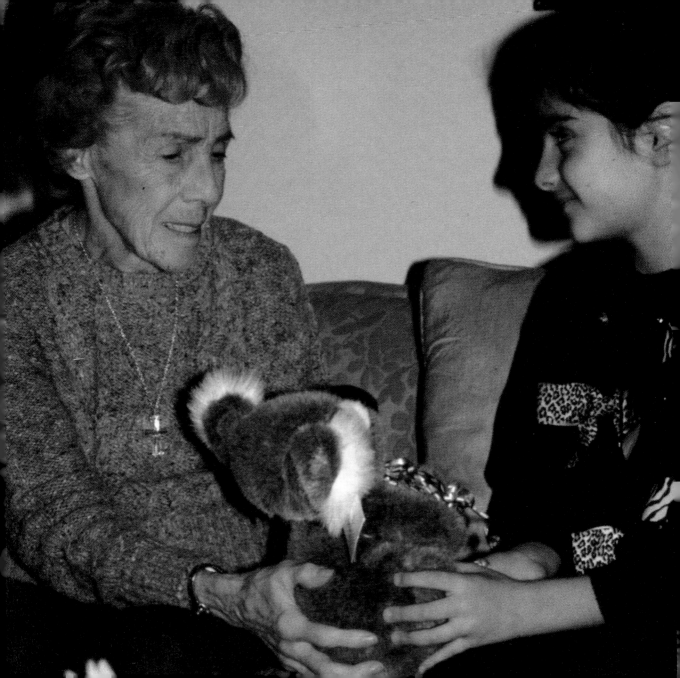

Kendra's Grandma

Every year, Kendra's grandma gave her a stuffed animal for her birthday. But Grandma was sick for Kendra's seventh birthday. After her birthday party, Kendra's mother gave her a cuddly koala bear. The card said, "Love, Grandma." But Kendra knew it wasn't from her. She had seen her mother wrapping it the night before.

◀ Grandma had always given Kendra a stuffed animal for her birthday.

What Is Alzheimer's Disease?

Kendra thought Grandma had forgotten about her. Her mother explained that she has a sickness called **Alzheimer's disease** (ALZ-hy-merz diz-EAZ). When a person has **AD** (AY-DEE), her brain doesn't work like everybody else's. Our brains send signals to our body parts, telling them what to do. When someone has AD, her brain mixes up those signals. But even though she can't remember everything she used to, Grandma still loves Kendra very much.

Kendra's mom explained that Kendra's ▶ grandma still loved her very much.

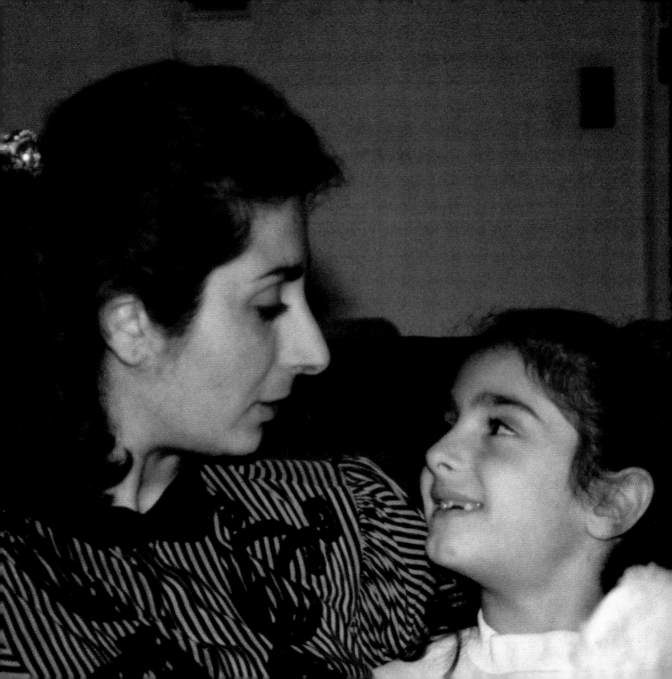

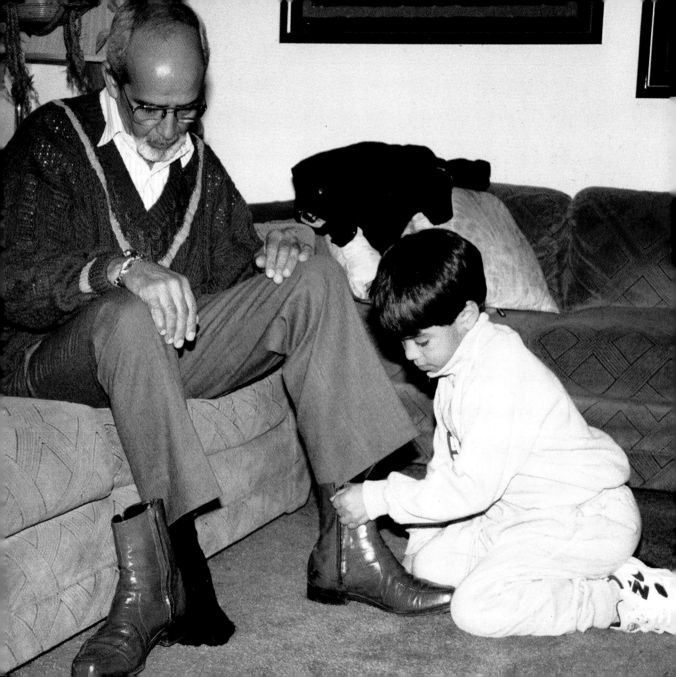

The Stages of Alzheimer's

At first, a person with AD forgets things like phone numbers. Not everyone who forgets things has AD. But everyone who has AD forgets things. After a few years, someone with AD may not even remember what a phone is for. Much later, a person with AD will seem very different. Your grandpa, or someone else you love, may call you by your mother's name. He may talk about his childhood as if it were yesterday.

◀ A person with AD may forget how to put on his shoes.

Taking Care of Someone with Alzheimer's

If your grandpa is in a later stage of AD, he probably has trouble with lots of things. He may forget to shut the water off after a shower. Or he may not remember that he has turned the oven on. He will need someone to help him. The grown-ups in your family will need to figure out who can best take care of him.

Your grandpa may not remember where he lives. ▶

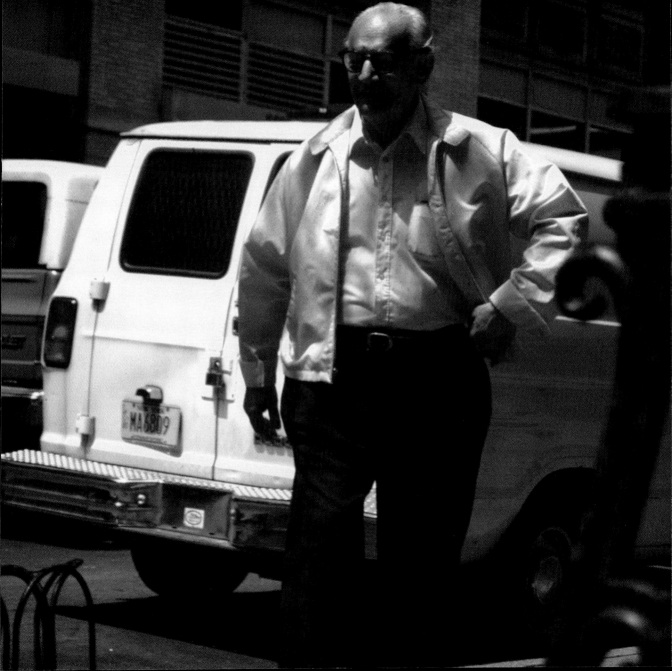

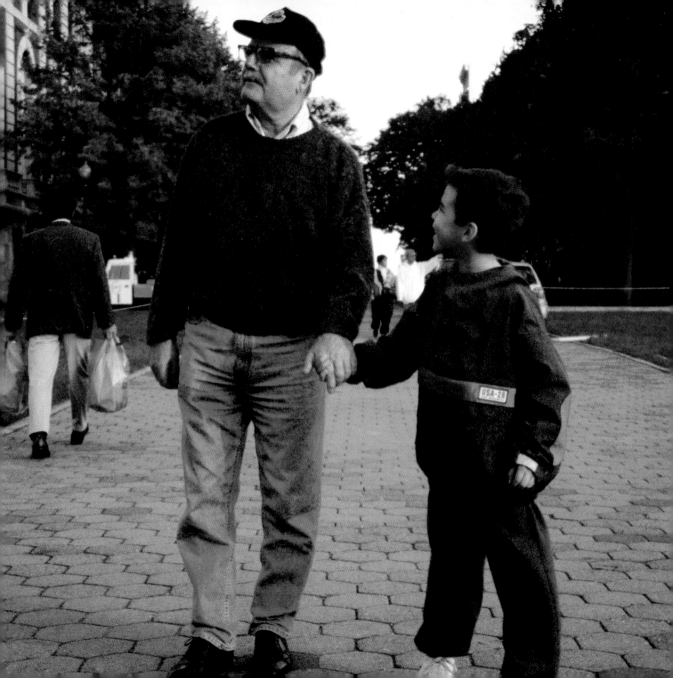

When Your Grandpa Moves In

Your parents may decide that Grandpa should move in with you. If this happens, you will have more chances to see how AD has changed your grandfather. He may ask you the same questions over and over. You may find him walking around a lot or talking to himself.

Try not to get angry with Grandpa. He can't help these changes in himself.

◀ You may find your grandpa wandering around outside.

Going to a Nursing Home

Sometimes a person with AD goes to a nursing home. People in nursing homes are taken care of by doctors and nurses. When you visit a nursing home you may notice that it smells like food, or perfume, or cleanser. You'll see some people in wheelchairs and some walking around. Others may be making strange noises or lying in bed. It may be scary to be around people who are sick. But remember—almost everyone you see there is somebody's grandma or grandpa.

14

Doctors and nurses can take good care of your grandma at a nursing home. ▶

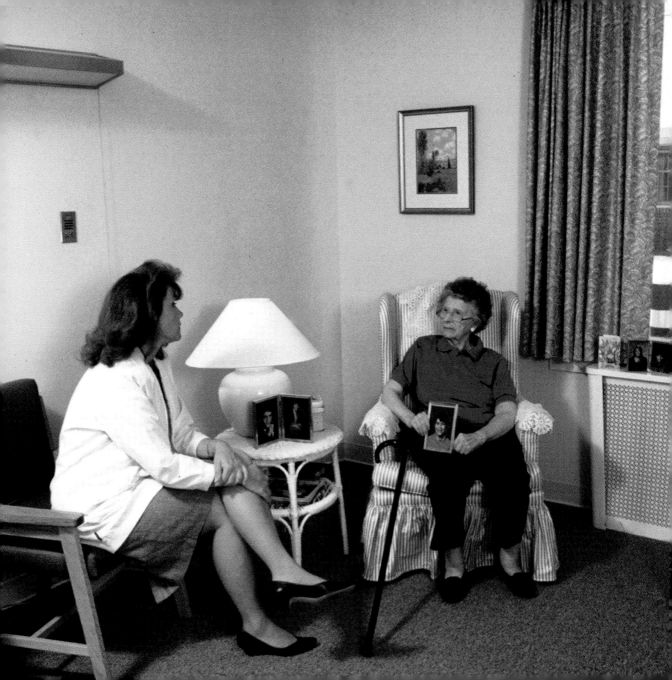

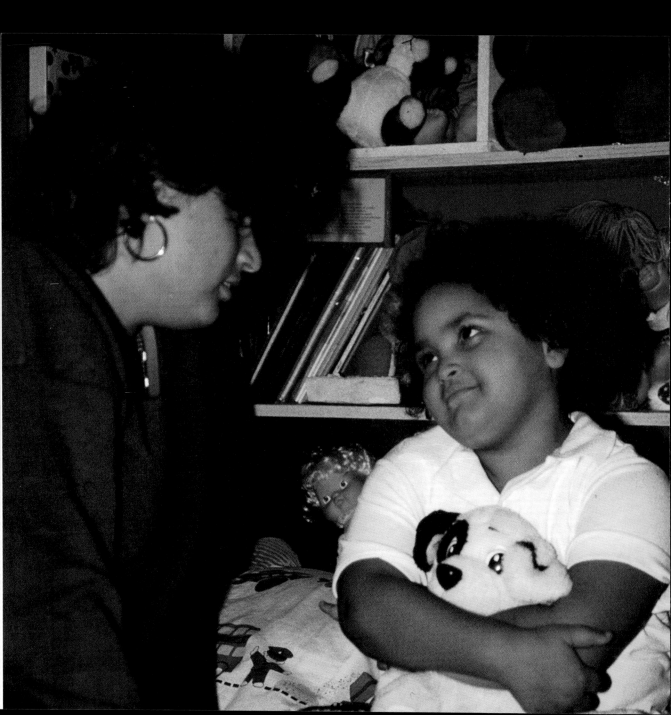

How Do You Feel?

You may feel scared or sad or angry about your grandma's change. *All* those feelings are normal. It's very hard to watch someone you love get sick. Your parents are probably feeling the same way. You may even notice them whispering to each other more than usual.

It's important that you talk to them about how you feel. They can help you understand that *nothing* you did changed Grandma.

◀ Talk to your parents about how you feel about the changes in Grandma.

You Can Help

But there is something you can do now.

You can love Grandma just as much as you did before she had AD. You can spend time with her, which will make her very happy even if she can't show it.

You can visit Grandma in the nursing home. Or sit with Grandma if she lives at home with you. You don't even have to talk. If you hold her hand and love her, she'll know.

You can help your grandma just ▶
by sitting with her.

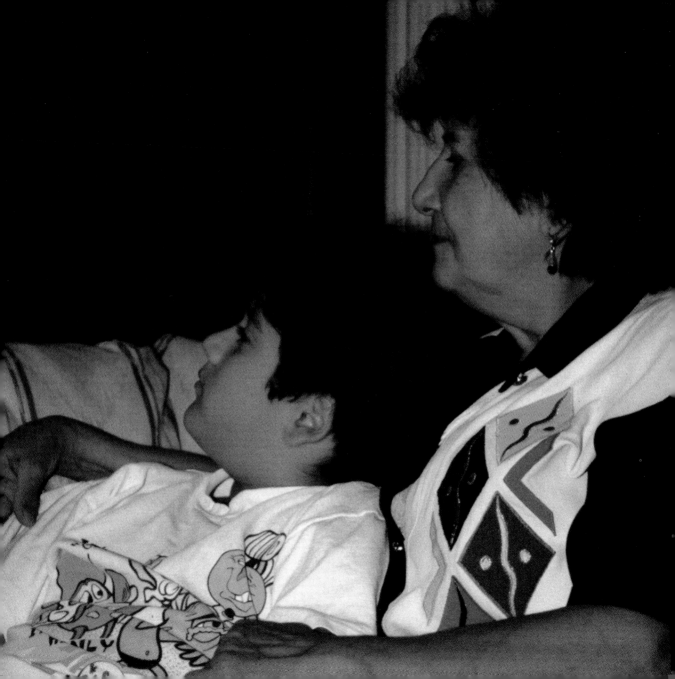

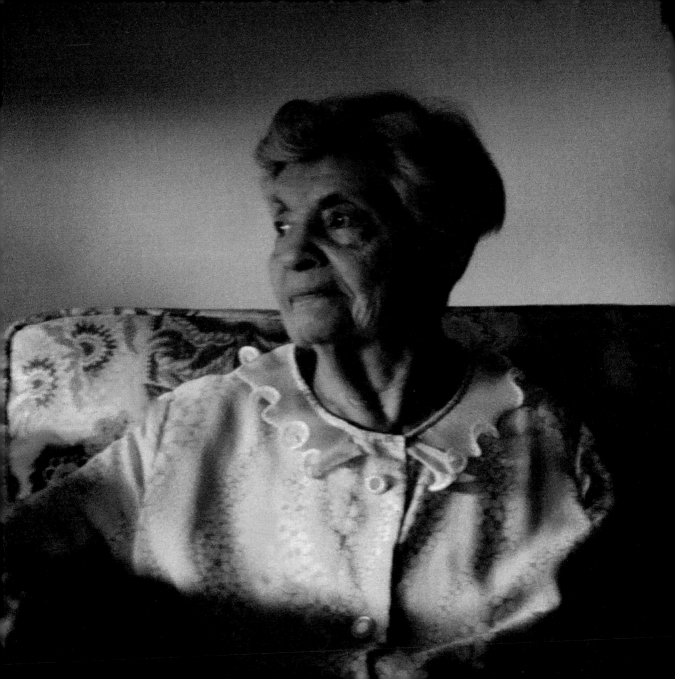

What's Going to Happen?

Having Alzheimer's isn't like having the flu or the chicken pox. Your grandma can't go to the doctor to get cured.

As your grandma gets older, you'll see more signs of AD. She may stop talking. And she may not show that she recognizes you.

Try to understand that she can't help this. If she could hug you and kiss you, and go for walks with you, she would.

◄ Try to remember that your grandma loves you even if she can't show you or tell you.

21

Don't Give Up

It's not easy to watch a person who has AD change. Everybody gets sad and confused about these changes—your parents, your sisters or brothers, even your grandma herself.

But your grandma will always be your grandma, no matter how she changes. She'll always love you, even if you can't always tell. And you can think of her the way she was, and continue to love her the way she is.

Glossary

Alzheimer's disease (ALZ-hy-merz diz-EAZ) An
  illness that affects a person's brain. It cannot
  be cured.

AD (AY-DEE) The abbreviation of Alzheimer's
  disease.

Index